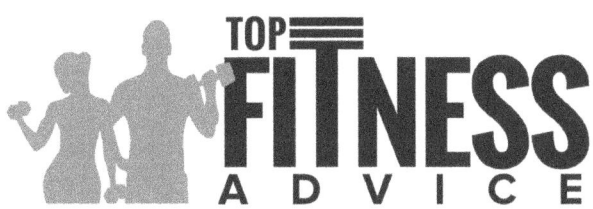

15 Minute Body Fix

3rd Edition

15-Minute Exercises & Workouts To Help Resize Your Thighs, Blast Belly Fat & Sculpt Lean Arms!

LINDA WESTWOOD

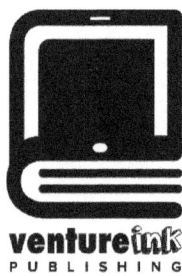

First published in 2015 by Venture Ink Publishing

Copyright © Top Fitness Advice 2019

All rights reserved.

No part of this book may be reproduced in any form without permission in writing from the author. No part of this publication may be reproduced or transmitted in any form or by any means, mechanic, electronic, photocopying, recording, by any storage or retrieval system, or transmitted by email without the permission in writing from the author and publisher.

Requests to the publisher for permission should be addressed to publishing@ventureink.co

For more information about the contents of this book or questions to the author, please contact Linda Westwood at linda@topfitnessadvice.com

Disclaimer

This book provides wellness management information in an informative and educational manner only, with information that is general in nature and that is not specific to you, the reader. The contents of this book are intended to assist you and other readers in your personal wellness efforts. Consult your physician regarding the applicability of any information provided in this book to you.

Nothing in this book should be construed as personal advice or diagnosis, and must not be used in this manner. The information provided about conditions is general in nature. This information does not cover all possible uses, actions, precautions, side-effects, or interactions of medicines, or medical procedures. The information in this book should not be considered as complete and does not cover all diseases, ailments, physical conditions, or their treatment.

You should consult with your physician before beginning any exercise, weight loss, or health care program. This book should not be used in place of a call or visit to a competent health-care professional. You should consult a health care professional before adopting any of the suggestions in this book or before drawing inferences from it.

Any decision regarding treatment and medication for your condition should be made with the advice and consultation of a qualified health care professional. If you have, or suspect you have, a health-care problem, then you should immediately contact a qualified health care professional for treatment.

No Warranties: The author and publisher don't guarantee or warrant the quality, accuracy, completeness, timeliness, appropriateness or suitability of the information in this book, or of any product or services referenced in this book.

The information in this book is provided on an "as is" basis and the author and publisher make no representations or warranties of any kind with respect to this information. This book may contain inaccuracies, typographical errors, or other errors.

Liability Disclaimer: The publisher, author, and other parties involved in the creation, production, provision of information, or delivery of this book specifically disclaim any responsibility, and shall not be held liable for any damages, claims, injuries, losses, liabilities, costs, or obligations including any direct, indirect, special, incidental, or consequences damages (collectively known as "Damages") whatsoever and howsoever caused, arising out of, or in connection with the use or misuse of the site and the information contained within it, whether such Damages arise in contract, tort, negligence, equity, statute law, or by way of other legal theory.

Table of Contents

Disclaimer	3
Who is this book for?	7
What will this book teach you?	9
Introduction	11
Chapter 1: What is the 15-Minute Body Fix?	15
Chapter 2: Let's Begin	21
Chapter 3: Full Body Fix	25
Chapter 4: Resize Your Thighs	39
Chapter 5: Blast Belly Fat	47
Chapter 6: Sculpt Lean Arms	51
Chapter 7: What You Should Eat	61
Breakfast	67
Lunch	73
Dinner	78
Chapter 8: Top Tips for Success	85
Conclusion	93
Final Words	95

Would you prefer to listen to my book, rather than read it?

Download the audiobook version for free!

If you go to the special link below and sign up to Audible as a new customer, you can get the audiobook version of my book completely free.

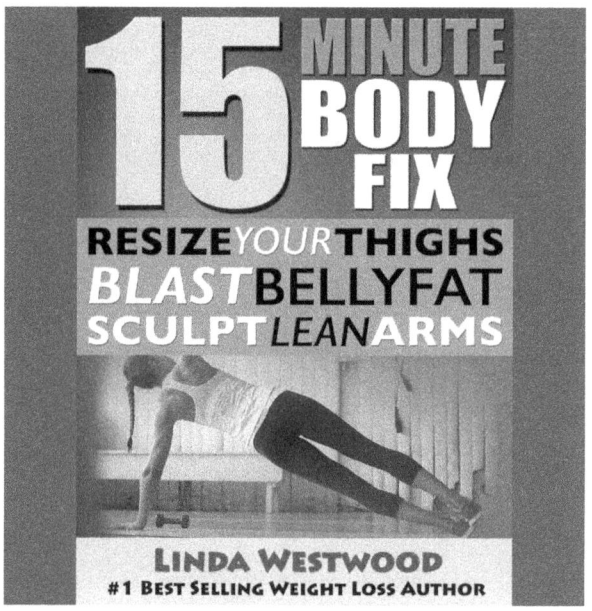

Go here to get your audiobook version for free:

TopFitnessAdvice.com/go/15Minute

Who is this book for?

Do you need a *strong* kick-start with your weight loss?

Are you ready to lose weight and transform your with just 15 minutes of exercise a day?

Or do you just wish that your diet would allow fat to just fall off *effortlessly?*

If you answered "Yes" to any of those questions – **this book is for you!**

I am going to share with you the most effective way to slim down, improve your health & have more energy than ever before. I will also teach you how you can start implementing weight training and why it's one of the key ingredients to faster weight loss. And if you eat right, you only have to work out 15 minutes a day!

I have put it all together in this awesome book – a special edition for women-only!

You can be a complete beginner or someone who works out regularly, it doesn't matter!

If this sounds like it could help you, then keep reading…

What will this book teach you?

Inside, I will teach you one of the best ways a woman can begin to transform her body, specifically targeting the belly, thighs and arms. These exercises and the diet plan will not only boost your weight loss, but also rejuvenate both your mind and body!

You will feel the healthiest you have ever felt – have the most energy you have ever had – and you will feel like the fat is just *melting away!*

How? Because you're going to be eating well, and doing some of the most effective workouts that accelerates body transformation in a short period of time.

In this book, I give you the exact plan that will change your life – all you have to do is follow it!

One of the most important things for you to realize when reading this book is that it *really does work!*

However…

For you to achieve *real success*, you HAVE to take action and apply it your life. Eat the right diet according to the plan I have set out, and follow the workouts and exercises.

This is where most people fail – they read through the entire book but do nothing. You MUST try your best to apply ras you read through the book!

Introduction

Physical fitness is paramount to health. Medical authorities agree it is impossible to be healthy without some degree of physical fitness. There are many definitions, but the simplest one is enough for us to understand what being "fit" really means – "a general state of well-being, as manifested in the ability to perform tasks related to sports, occupations, or daily life without undue stress".

The key here is that it's a "state" – meaning we can achieve the state of being "physically fit". And this is achieved through a healthy diet and moderate exercise. It's basically "maintenance" of your body. Just like you would invest time and money to invest your car (if it were broken or not running efficiently, you need to maintain your body.

However, according to the United States Centers for Disease Control, 80 percent of adult Americans do not get the recommended amount of exercise per week.

Although some countries are certainly fitter than others, people all over the world now seem to be less concerned with their health than they should be.

Why is this happening? If we are concerned about our health, why aren't we exercising enough?

Well, many people have misunderstandings around exercise and fitness, especially on what is "enough" or what activity can be considered an adequate amount of exercise per day.

One such misconception is the matter of "time". Many experts say that at least 30 minutes of exercise daily is optimum for health and fitness. You can find this recommendation posted in magazines, newspapers, and everywhere online.

But there is a problem with this. Firstly, along with this recommendation you will commonly see these "experts" advising that something as simple as walking is counted toward this 30 minutes per day of exercise.

Does this mean that everyone who walks 30 minutes per day (spread out throughout the day) is exercising enough? Exercising enough to lose weight, maintain a healthy weight, or achieve optimal fitness levels? This is where the problems begin. It is simply wrong. Most of us do walk upwards of 30 minutes per day in our regular day (at work, at school, or with the kids). This is not enough.

Secondly, the so-called "expert" exercise recommendations do take into account that in today's age we are working longer hours, and multi-tasking more than ever before. We are always squeezing more into every day, especially if we have kids, a job, a large family, and other activities or hobbies.

So, here's what I propose to you (it's my mission is on this planet, it's what I believe, and it's what I will teach you in this book)...

I know, for a fact, that we can get an adequate amount of exercise in just 15 minutes per day. How? By performing specific workouts each day, so that over the course of a week we have targeted various muscle groups, increased our heart rates in each workout, and most importantly combined all of this hard work with an optimized diet to accelerate weight loss, maintain or grow muscle, and tremendously improved our health and energy levels. This is achieving the state of being "physically fit".

This means that my workouts are designed for maximum results in a minimal amount of time. Combining muscle training with quick repetition means a cardiovascular workout is often included as well as toning and improving muscle strength.

The term "healthy eating" covers a broad range of subjects. At the moment, it is also quite a controversial term. The only thing that the experts seem to agree on is that they disagree about what "healthy eating" consists of.

Now, that's all good and well but it doesn't help you out if you want to learn how to supercharge your nutrition. If you really want to get your body firing on all cylinders, you need the right nutrition information and you need it now. And you don't want to have to sort through all the confusing data out there.

Not to worry – I have done that for you. I have laid out a simple plan that is proven to be effective.

With my experience in the field of physical fitness, I have zeroed in on what works when you need to perform at a higher level.

And it's not all about starving yourself or eating foods that you really cannot stand. It's not about isolating yourself from your friends for fear of a few bites of junk food.

What it is about is making the right food choices. And with this book, this will be easy for you.

I've made it as simple as possible. I give you lists of foods that you should concentrate on. I've scrapped calorie counting – it's not effective anyway – and concentrated on giving you food that is naturally nutritious and wholesome. This plan will help you relearn how to trust your own body and its natural hunger signals.

You have a 7-day meal plan to get you started.

Want to take it up a notch? Read about the power foods that boost your health and energy levels.

Learn which foods to eat to boost your body's own fat-blasting systems. The basic plan is simple, the recipes provided taste great.

Are you ready to turn your body into a lean, mean, fat-blasting machine?

Lastly, many people believe that they must join a gym to be successful. Although a gym may be necessary for some wishing to learn specialized routines or use specific equipment, it is not required to work on fitness, especially at the beginner level.

The 15 Minute Body Fix method is designed to shatter those myths, get you moving and propel you forward to fitness!

Chapter 1

What is the 15-Minute Body Fix?

Work Smarter, Not Harder

Time management is the ability to work smarter, not harder. This skill is extremely important into today's increasingly complex world. If the average person is to fit in work, family, and entertainment, much less exercise, planning is essential. This is where the 15-Minute Body Fix comes in.

The 15-Minute Body Fix is a fitness plan that anyone can fit into his or her lives. It is based upon a series of workouts, targeted for specific zones of the body. Not only will they help you to be fit, but you will sculpt your body, and lose inches. Weight loss is a natural side effect of exercise, so if you are consistent, the 15-minute Body Fix can assist you with that goal as well.

You will find workouts here for total body fitness, and some that are specifically targeted for problem areas: your thighs, your belly, and your arms. The total body workouts can be alternated with the targeted ones, focusing on the zones you feel need work.

For example, the total body workout could be done 3 days a week, with zone workouts in between, with whatever emphasis you decide is most important for you. As we will discuss in more detail, you should not do targeted workouts on the same area two days in a row. Mix it up!

A Healthier Lifestyle

Adding more exercise to your life can only benefit you, provided you exercise safely as discussed in more detail in the next chapter. However, if you are working out to lose weight in addition to becoming more physically fit, you will need to make changes to your diet as well.

The 15-Minute Body Fix will work best when accompanied by these changes. Observing portion sizes, choosing foods that are more nutritious, and limiting sugar, starch and alcohol will improve your health and the effectiveness of your workout.

Be aware, it's not necessary to change radically all aspects of your life at once. In fact, this can sabotage your plans before you really get started by overwhelming your system. Add elements of the 15-Minute Body Fix gradually to your life, and continue adding consistently until you are meeting your final goal.

All You Need Is You

A common complaint about beginning a fitness routine is expense: extensive equipment and videos to buy, or a pricey gym membership. All the workouts in the 15-Minute Body Fix are specifically chose to require little more equipment than your body weight.

Body weight workouts are designed to use your own weight instead of a dumbbell. These kinds of exercises place your body in what is called a disadvantaged position, requiring more strength to make the move. Pushups are the most famous of these exercises, but there are many more. These workouts also usually require the use of several muscle groups, so even if they are zone targeted, you will still continue to strengthen your other parts.

If any other equipment is involved, it will be a common household item, like a towel or a chair. You may also need to use a wall stabilize yourself. You will need a timer. However, a common kitchen timer will do, as will the stopwatch function on most cell phones. No fancy fitness equipment is needed for the 15-Minute Body Fix.

Discover Scientifically-Proven "Shortcuts" & "Hacks" to Lose Weight FASTER (With Very Little Effort)

For this month only, you can get Linda's best-selling & most popular book absolutely free – *Weight Loss Secrets You NEED to Know.*

Get Your FREE Copy Here:
TopFitnessAdvice.com/Bonus

Discover scientifically-proven tips to help you lose weight faster and easier than ever before. With this book, readers were able to improve their weight loss results and fitness levels. So, it's highly recommended that you get this book, especially while it's free!

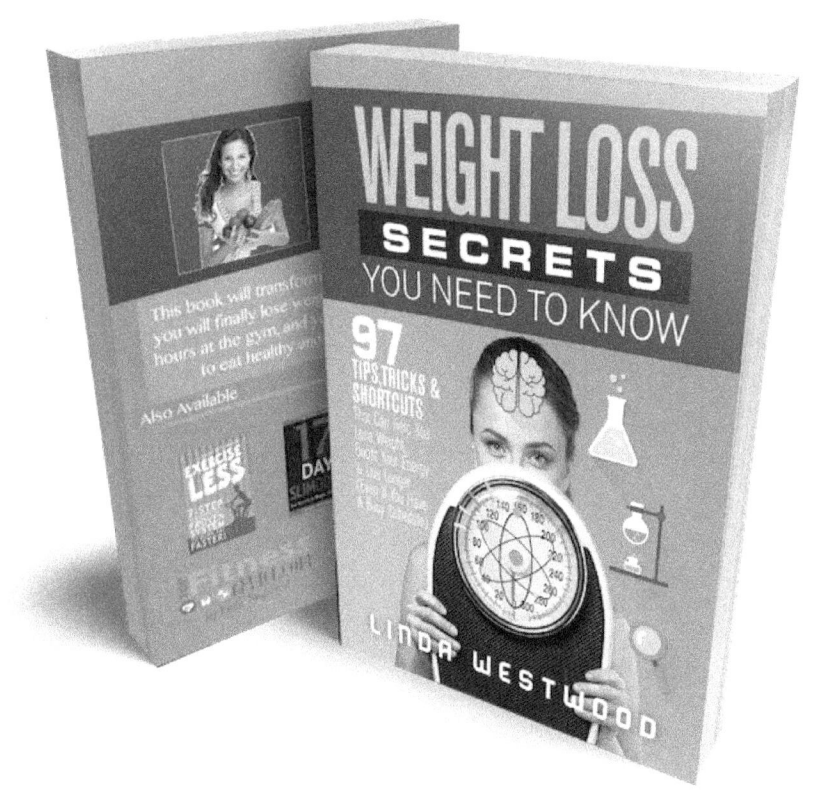

Get Your FREE Copy Here:

TopFitnessAdvice.com/Bonus

Chapter 2

Let's Begin

Safety First

You will often hear the advice to have a check-up with your doctor prior to beginning any exercise plan. This is an excellent idea, but it should also emphasize to you the importance of safety in your planning. So how do you go about getting started safely?

First, how many days a week do you plan to work out. Experts advise at least one day of rest from organized exercise each week. Judge this by your current fitness level. For example, if you currently don't exercise at all, you may want to start with three days a week and work up to a more strenuous plan.

Next, decide what body zones you most need to focus on. Will you sculpt your arms two days, and blast your belly fat for one, or vice versa? If you are starting slow, you may only be able to fit in one targeted workout per week to start.

Stretch It Out

Make time to stretch prior to your workout. The American Academy of Sports Medicine advises stretching prior to exercise. Stretching improves flexibility, and helps prevent muscle injury. However, there is no proven benefit to extended stretching time.

People tend to naturally stretch after sleeping, and sitting for extended periods of time. So, your body already knows the benefits of stretching.

Here are a few stretches that can help you prepare for exercise:

Standing Cat-Camel

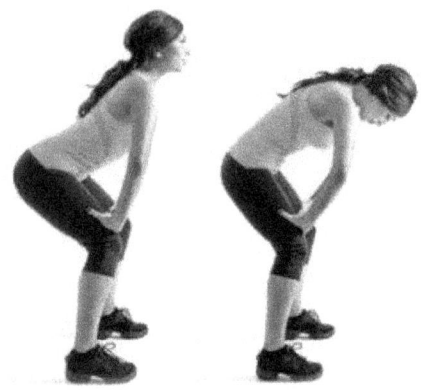

1. Stand with your feet shoulder width apart and your knees slightly bent.

2. Lean forward, placing your hands just above your knees.

3. Stretch your back into a rounded shape, closing off your chest and curving your shoulders forward.

4. Then arch your back, opening your chest and throwing your shoulders back.

Scissor Hamstring Stretch

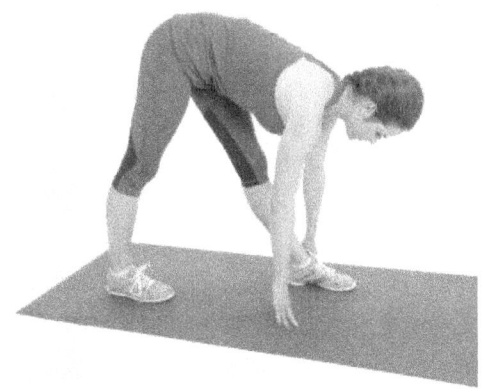

1. Stand with your feet together. Step back about two feet in distance with one of your feet.

2. Bend forward from your hips. Keep your back straight.

3. Keep your legs straight. Hold briefly. Switch sides.

Bicep Wall Stretch

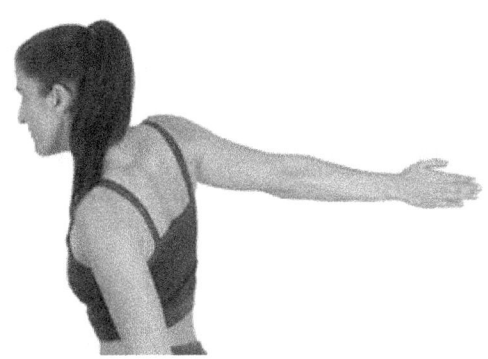

1. Place the palm, shoulder and inner elbow of one of your arms against the wall.

2. Keeping in contact with the wall, turn your body slowly away from it. You should feel the stretch in your arm muscles and your chest.

You may add other stretches as you add workout days if you feel you need them.

I hope that you are enjoying this book so far, and if you could spare 30 seconds, I would greatly appreciate you leaving a review on Amazon.com.

Chapter 3

Full Body Fix

Full Body Workouts

15-minute workouts can include the entire body, and there are many benefits to this approach. Obviously, the time savings is important, but what are the other benefits you can expect?

You will burn more calories than you do with workouts that target specific areas. The compound exercises in a full body workout require your major muscle groups to work together. This expends more energy to coordinate, which in turn uses up more calories.

You will build more muscle, as well, as you would using an isolated approach. Although this seems to be counterintuitive, some fitness instructors assert that one day a week's heavy concentration on one area is not enough work for most people to achieve muscle growth. The consistency of a total body workout done several days during the week is more effective.

You will maximize your workout's efficiency. Using several muscles together as you will in a full body workout, the muscles are worked just as hard as they would be during a much more extensive time on multiple machines. Pay attention to doing each move as perfectly as possible.

Full Body Workout #1

Set your timer to 15 minutes. This is what is called a circuit workout, which is to say that once you have completed the exercises, you will simply start them over again.

Begin with ten pushups. **Pushups** are done correctly as described:

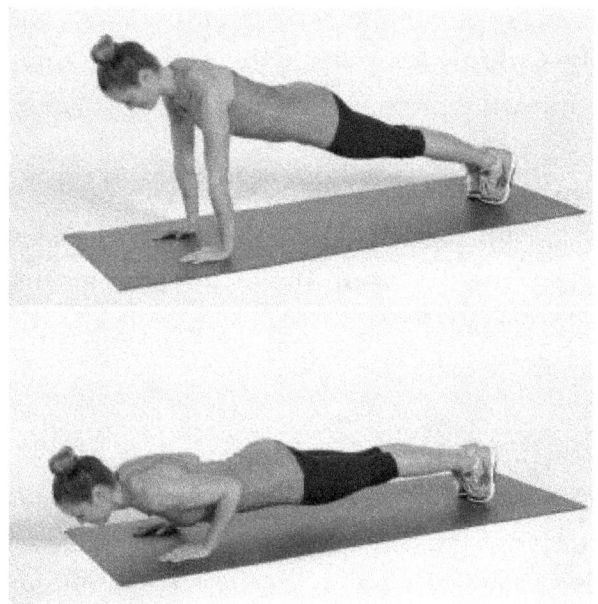

1. Place your hands right under your shoulders.

2. Position your feet, on your toes, at hip width apart.

3. Place the body in a plank position, that is to say, your body should be in a straight line from your heels, through your hips, to the back of your head.

4. Keep your neck neutral, keeping it in line with your shoulders.

5. Lower your body with your arms, as low as you can go to the ground while maintaining control, and keeping your elbows close to your body.

6. Do not let your body out of that planking position even if it slows you down. You may widen the set of your feet to assist your stability if absolutely necessary.

7. If this position is impossible for you to maintain in the beginning, you may want to do pushups resting on your knees rather than your toes. It is still important to keep your back straight.

8. Raise yourself to the original position.

Do Jumping Jacks for the remainder of minute 1.

Jumping Jacks are performed this way:

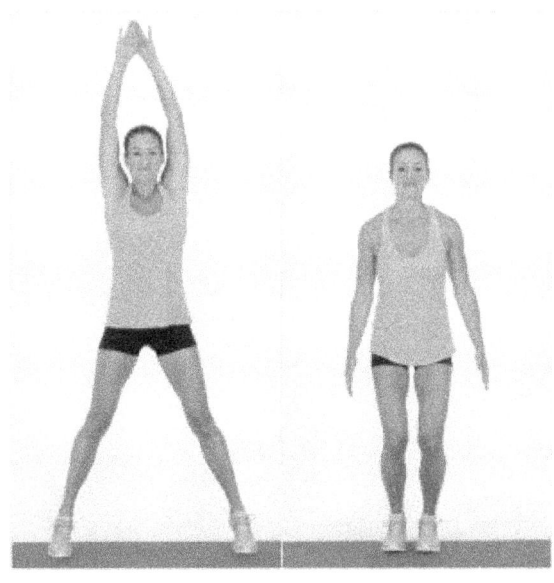

1. Begin in an erect position, your arms at your sides, and your feet together.

2. Bend your knees just a little, and propel yourself into the air, about 2 inches up.

3. While you are in the air, move your legs out to the side to at least shoulder width, although you can go wider.

4. At the same time, you will be moving your slightly bent arms over your head, to meet above your head as you land.

5. Upon landing, immediately jump back to your original erect positions.

At minute 1, do 10 Spider Lunges.

Spider Lunges are accomplished according to the following directions:

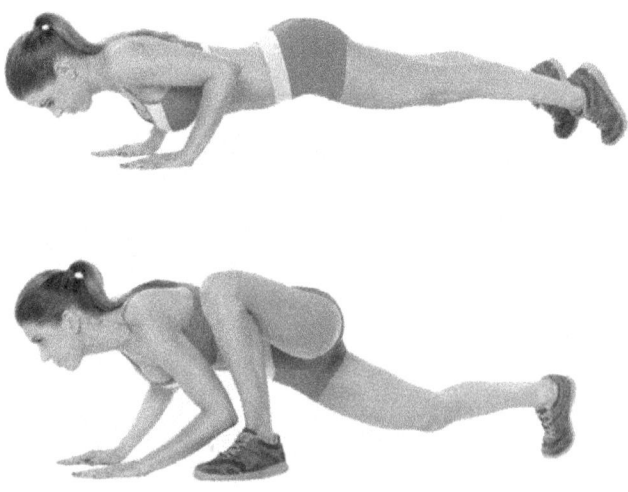

1. Begin in plank position, as with a push up.

2. Move your right foot to the outside of your right hand.

3. Set your foot down flat.

4. Then, move your foot back to the starting position.

5. Repeat on the other foot.

6. Make sure you remain in plank position, throughout.

Do Jumping Jacks until the timer reads minute 2. Follow the above direction for Jumping Jacks.

At minute 2, do 10 Jumping Lunges.

Jumping Lunges are done this way:

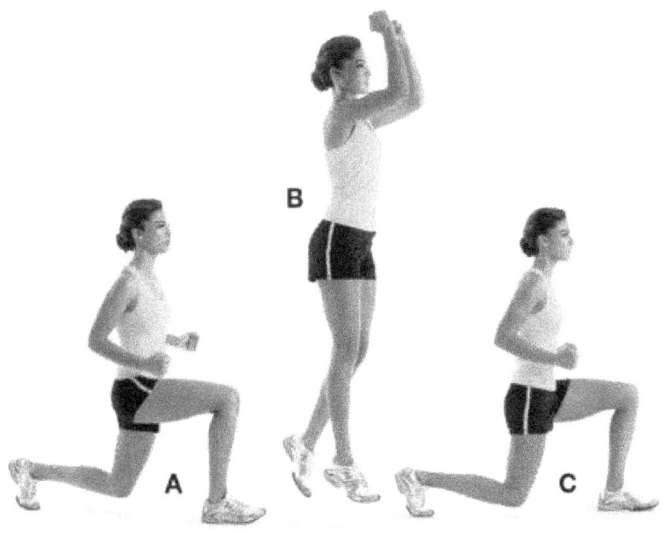

1. From a standing position, step forward with one foot.

2. Bend the knee of the front foot to 90 degrees.

3. At the same time, bend the back leg as if you are going to place it on the floor.

4. Keep your back vertical throughout the exercise.

5. Go as low as your flexibility allows without actually placing your back knee on the floor. *This is a standard lunge, and depending on your current physical condition, you may need to stop there, and work up to the jumping lunge.*

6. Your arm should pump forward slightly bent, as when running, while you lunge, and your arms should switch when you switch feet.

7. To switch feet, use your leg muscles to propel yourself upward into a jump, while switching the position of your legs.

8. Land into a lunge with the opposite foot in front.

Do Jumping Jacks until minute 3.
At minute 3, do 10 Walkouts.

Walkouts are performed this way:

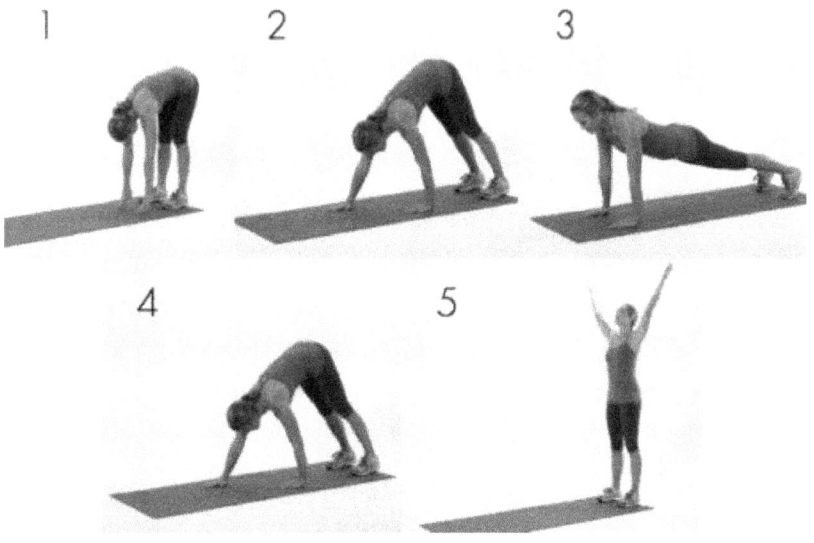

1. Stand with legs apart at shoulder width.

2. Keeping your back straight, bend over and place your hands on the floor.

3. Bend your knees as little as your flexibility will allow. Eventually you will be able to perform this with your legs straight.

4. "Walk" your hands forward, maintaining a tight core for stability, until you are in a plank position.

5. "Walk" your hands back to the front of your feet.

6. Push your hips as high as possible and press your heels into the floor as you "walk" back.

7. Return to a standing position.

Do Jumping Jacks until minute 4.

At minute 4, REPEAT the steps listed above until your 15 minutes are up.

As with the exercises, there are some accommodations for a beginning fitness level. You may wish to start with 5 repetitions of exercises, filling in the rest of the minute with Jumping Jacks. You may include a rest between cycles from 45 seconds to 1.5 minutes.

Full Body Workout #2

This workout is broken into two parts, listed here as A and B. It is intended for you to do these repetitions as quickly as you are safely able to do so. You may continue to cycle between Part A and B for 15 minutes when you can speed them up.

Part A

1. Do 10 Jumping Lunges.
2. Do 10 Spider Lunges.
3. Repeat this 8 times.
4. Rest 2 minutes.

Part B

1. Do 10 Pushups.
2. Do 10 Walkouts.
3. Repeat this 8 times.
4. Rest 2 minutes.

Full Body Workout #3

This workout is performed in a similar fashion to Workout #1, in that you fill in your minute with Jumping Jacks. Any new exercises will be explained as above.

Begin with 10 Plank Taps. **Plank Taps** are performed this way:

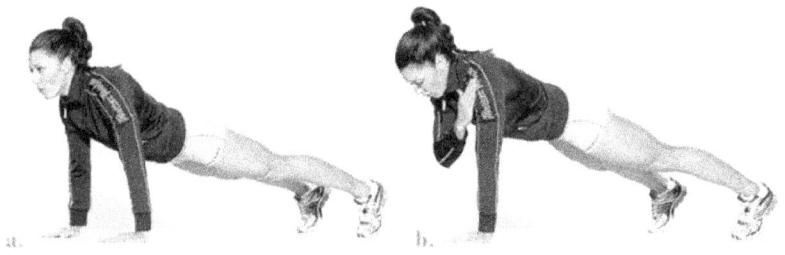

1. Begin in plank position.

2. Maintaining your form, reach up with your right hand and lightly tap your left shoulder.

3. Use all of your muscles to maintain your position while you tap.

4. Do not allow your weight to shift while you are tapping your shoulder. Focus on your other muscles holding the position.

5. Return your hand to the plank position.

Do Jumping Jacks until you complete minute 1.

If the plank tap is too difficult in the beginning, you may hold the plank position for 30 seconds and do Jumping Jacks for the other 30 seconds.

At minute 2, do 10 Squats. Squats are done safely this way:

1. Stand with your feet shoulder width apart. When you do the exercise, you may need to move them in to help you stay stable. Try one and adjust to remain safe before doing multiple repetitions.

2. Turn out your feet slightly, to help you maintain balance as you squat. You may adjust the angle of your feet to help you with stability.

3. Keep your chest open. Look slightly up and straight ahead.

4. Squat as deeply as flexibility and balance allow. For safety, make sure that your knees do not go past your toes as you squat. You may adjust the depth of your squat as your fitness level improves.

5. Keep your feet flat. Do not raise your heels or shift your weight onto your toes.
6. As you squat, bend your arms and bring your hands together in the middle of your chest, keeping your elbows aligned with your shoulders.

7. Return to an upright position.

Do Jumping Jacks to complete minute 2.

At minute 3, do 10 Side Lunges. **Side Lunges** are performed correctly this way:

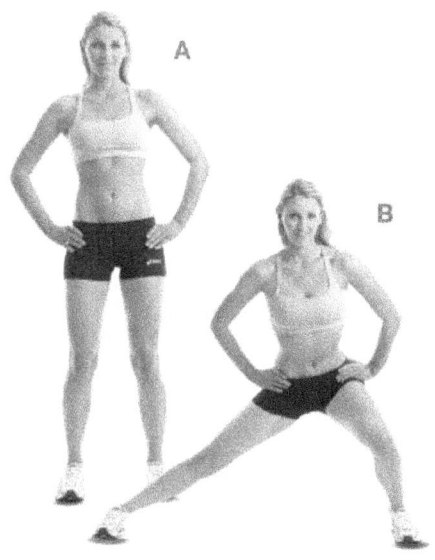

1. Begin in a standing position with your feet together. Clasp your hands in front of your chest in a similar fashion as when you do squats. Step out to the side with your right foot as far as you comfortably can, and adjust this as you try the exercise so that you maintain balance and stability.

2. Keep your chest open.

3. Bend your right knee to lunge as low as flexibility and balance will allow. Shift your weight through your mid-foot and heel, not forward on your toes. Do not allow your knee to go past your toe.

Do Jumping Jacks to complete minute 3.

At minute 4, repeat the cycle through your 15 minutes.

Full Body Workout #4

Workout #4 is organized like Workout #2, with a Part A and a Part B. As a reminder, you should perform these exercises as quickly as you can, with respect to safety and form.

Part A

Begin with 10 Reverse Lunges. **Reverse Lunges** are accomplished correctly this way:

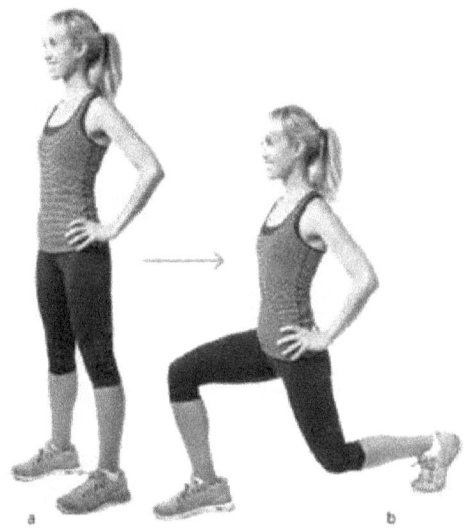

1. Start in a standing position, feet together, arms by your side.

2. Step back with your left foot. Keep your weight balanced between your feet.

3. Keep your chest open.

4. Pump your slightly bent left arm forward, fist moving up to stop at shoulder height.

5. Bend your knees slowly, until your right leg is at a 90 degree angle. Do not allow your weight to shift in your right leg toward the toe, and do not let your knee go beyond your toe.

6. Your left leg should lightly touch the floor. Be careful that your right knee does not buckle inward.

7. Push through your right heel as you stand up.

Do 10 Side Lunges.
Complete Part A 8 times.
Rest 2 minutes.

Part B

Do 10 Plank Taps.
Do 10 Pushups.
Complete Part B 8 times.
Rest 2 minutes.
Continue cycling this way for 15 minutes.

Full Body Workout #5

This workout is structured similarly to Workout #1 and #3. However, instead of Jumping Jacks to finish out your minute, you will simply run in place.

To begin, do 10 Walkouts.
Run in place to complete your minute.
At minute 1, do 10 Side Lunges.
Run in place to complete your minute.
At minute 2, do 10 Pushups.
Run in place to complete your minute.
At minute 3, do 10 Reverse Lunges.
Run in place to complete your minute.
At minute 4, REPEAT the steps listed above until your 15 minutes are up.

Chapter 4

Resize Your Thighs

These workouts will focus on your thighs and legs. Although your Full Body Workouts work these muscles, if this is a trouble spot for you in terms of strength, you may want a more targeted routine.

Leg and Thigh Workout #1

This workout is structured as others you have done, organized into Part A and Part B. You will be learning some new exercises, and using some you have already learned.

Part A

Do 10 Squat Jumps. **Squat Jumps** are performed safely this way:

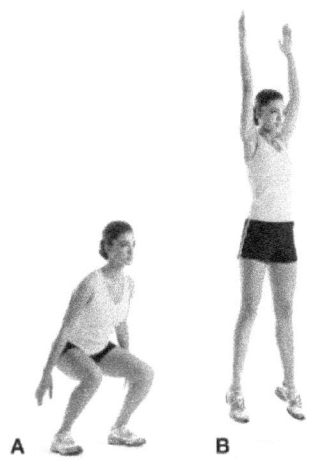

1. Squat until your thighs are parallel with the floor. Observe the safe squatting techniques you have already learned with squats, including not shifting your weight to your toes, and not allowing your knees to go past your toes.

2. Keep your chest open, your head slightly up and facing forward.

3. As you squat, bring your arms together till your hands clap.

4. From this position, jump as high as you can.

5. Push your arms behind you as you jump.

Do 10 Side Lunges.

Complete Part A 8 times.

Rest 2 minutes.

Part B

Do 10 Jumping Lunges.

Do 10 Glute Bridges. This is how to do **Glute Bridges:**

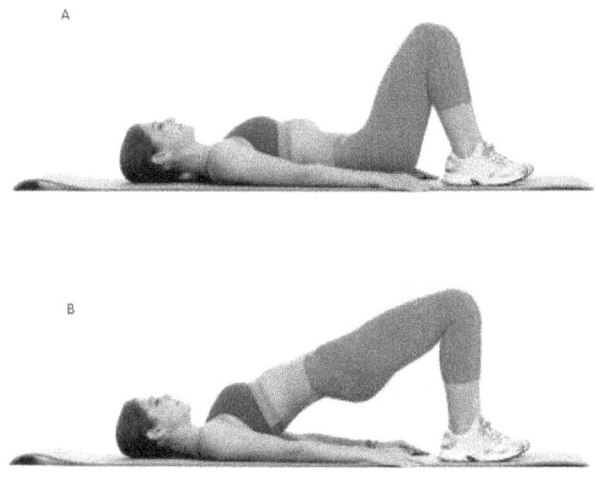

1. Lie in neutral position on your back on the floor. A neutral position is not totally flat, nor totally arched. You should be able to slip you hand part way into the curve of your back, but it should not fit all the way.

2. Place your feet, at hip width, evenly on the floor, with your toes pointing forward and your knees bent.

3. Contract your abdominal muscles. Imagine your belly button pulling in toward your spine. Keep your muscles this way throughout the exercise.

4. Push your hips up through your heels. You back should remain in the neutral position. If you back begins to arch or you feel pressure on your neck, you have done too fat.

5. You will keep your abdominals contracted as you lower your hips to the floor.

6. You should not truly rest in between repetitions, only lightly touch the floor.

Complete Part B 8 times.
Rest 2 minutes.
Continue cycling through Parts A and B for 15 minutes.

Leg and Thigh Workout #2

This workout is organized as a circuit. This means that you go from one exercise to another with only a 10 second rest in between. You are measuring by time instead of repetitions, so do each move as quickly and correctly as you can.

Do Squats for 30 seconds
Rest for 10 seconds.

Do Single-Leg Deadlifts for 30 seconds. The **Single-Leg Deadlift** is performed properly this way:

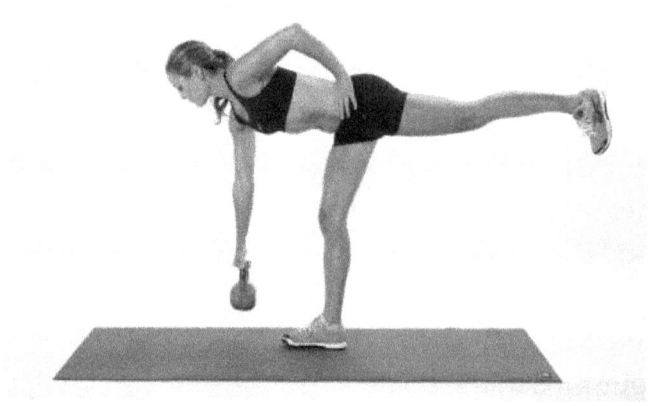

1. Begin in a standing position.

2. Raise one leg straight behind you with your toes pointing downwards.

3. As you raise your leg, bend forward from the hips, keeping your back flat. Keep your neck aligned with your spine, and loose, not tensed.

4. Your hands will be perpendicular to your chest. Do not reach towards the floor, as this may cause you to round your back.

5. Bend only as far as flexibility will allow, while keeping your core tight and your back straight.

6. Continue with your abs tight and your back straight as you lower your leg and return to a standing position.

7. Do not alternate legs until the next circuit. Stick with the single leg.

Rest 10 seconds.
Do Glute Bridges for 30 seconds.
Rest for 1 minute.

Repeat circuit for the entire 15 minutes. If you can only do a few exercises in the 30 seconds, do not get discouraged. You will get faster.

Lower Body Workout #3

This workout follows the pattern, which should now be familiar to you, of 10 repetitions and Jumping Jacks in between.

Begin with 10 Reverse Lunges.
Then do Jumping Jacks until your timer says 1 minute has passed.
At minute 1, do 10 Side Lunges.
Do Jumping Jacks until minute 2.
At minute 2, Do 10 Squats.
Do Jumping Jacks until minute 3.
At minute 3, do 10 Single-Leg Deadlifts.
Do Jumping Jacks until minute 4.
At minute 4, start again.
Do not forget to switch legs on your Single-Leg Deadlifts when you get there.

Leg and Thigh Workout #4

This workout will follow the established pattern with Part A and Part B.

Part A

1. Do 10 Jumping Lunges.
2. Rest 10 seconds.
3. Do 10 Single-Leg Deadlifts.
4. Rest 10 seconds.
5. Repeat Part A 8 times.

Part B

1. Do 10 Glute Bridges.

2. Rest 10 seconds.
3. Do 10 Squats.
4. Rest 10 seconds.
5. Repeat Part B 8 times.
6. Cycle between Parts A for the remainder of 15 minutes.

Leg and Thigh Workout #5

This workout is organized as a circuit.

1. Begin with 30 seconds of Jumping Lunges.
2. Rest 10 seconds.
3. Then, do 30 second of Reverse Lunges.
4. Rest 10 seconds.
5. Next, do 30 seconds of Squat Jumps.
6. Rest 1 minute.

Repeat this circuit as many times as you can in 15 minutes.

Once again, thank you for reading this book, and I hope you're getting a lot of valuable information. I would greatly appreciate it if you could take 30 seconds to leave me a review for this book on Amazon.com.

Enjoying this book?

Check out my other best sellers!

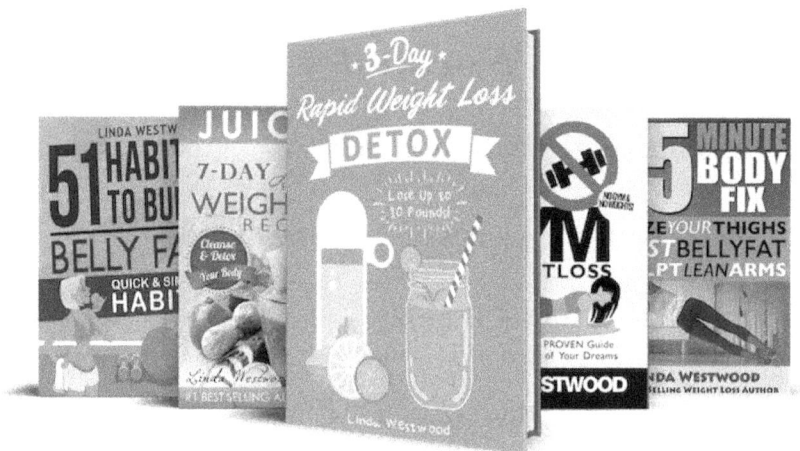

Get your next book on sale here:

TopFitnessAdvice.com/go/books

Chapter 5

Blast Belly Fat

Ah, that troublesome tummy! If you are imagining hundreds of sit-ups, think again. Many of the exercises we have already learned work our core abdominal muscles, and the workouts below will combine them perfectly to blast that belly fat in just 15 minutes!

Belly Blast Workout #1

This workout is organized as a circuit. Each exercise should be done in perfect form but as quickly as possible.

1. First, do Spider Lunges for 30 seconds.
2. Rest 10 seconds.
3. Then do Side Lunges for 30 seconds.
4. Rest 10 seconds.
5. Next, you will maintain a Plank position for 30 second. **The Plank** position has been used for many exercises you have learned, but all by itself it is a powerful tool for abdominal training. To review, when you plank, you hold yourself up by your arms and your toes. You keep your body in a straight line. That's it! It is harder simply to hold the position than you may think.
6. Rest 1 minute.

You will repeat this circuit as many times as you can in 15 minutes. The number of repetitions you do depends on you, and you can always speed yourself up.

Belly Blast Workout #2

This workout is based upon the 10 repetitions, Jumping Jacks pattern, optimized to strengthen your abdominal muscles.

1. Begin with 10 Plank Taps.
2. Then do Jumping Jacks to fill minute 1.
3. At the 1 minute mark, do 10 Walkouts.
4. Do Jumping Jacks for 2 minutes.
5. When your timer says 2 minutes, do 10 Single-Leg Deadlifts.
6. Fill the rest of minute 3 with Jumping Jacks.
7. When you get to minute 3 on your timer, do 10 jumping lunges.
8. Follow them with Jumping Jacks till your timer gets to 4 minutes.
9. Then repeat the cycle.

Remember to switch legs on your Single-Leg Deadlifts whenever the cycle starts over.

Belly Blast Workout #3

This workout is a Part A and B cycle.

Part A

1. Start with 10 Plank Taps.
2. Rest 10 seconds.
3. Move to 10 Jumping Lunges.
4. Rest 10 seconds.
5. Repeat this pattern 8 times.

Part B

1. Do 10 Spider Lunges.
2. Rest 10 seconds.
3. Do 10 Reverse Lunges.
4. Rest 10 seconds.
5. Repeat Part B 8 times.

Rest 1 minute, and then start again with Part A.

Continue this for the remainder of 15 minutes.

Belly Blast Workout #4

1. Begin with 10 Walkouts.
2. Then, run in place for the remainder of minute 1.
3. When the timer reaches 1 minute, do 10 reverse lunges.
4. Run in place until the timer reaches 2 minutes.
5. At 2 minutes, do 10 Spider Lunges.
6. Run in place until the timer reaches 3 minutes.
7. Then assume the Plank Position, and hold it for 30 seconds.
8. Use the other 30 seconds of minute 3 for running in place.

Belly Blast Workout #5

1. Do Plank Taps for 30 seconds.
2. Rest 10 seconds.
3. Do Single-Leg Deadlifts for 30 seconds.
4. Rest 10 seconds.
5. Do Walkouts for 30 seconds.
6. Rest 1 minute.

7. Repeat circuit for the remainder of 15 minutes.

Chapter 6

Sculpt Lean Arms

Although many of the exercises you have already learned are helpful to tone your arms and improve upper body strength, you will be introduced to some new moves for these workouts.

The formats will continue to be familiar ones.

Lean Arm Workout #1

This is a circuit workout.

1. Start with Pushups for 30 seconds.
2. Rest for 10 seconds.
3. Do Plank Taps for 30 seconds.
4. Rest for 10 seconds.
5. Do Walkouts for 30 seconds.
6. Rest for 1 minute.
7. Repeat circuit until 15 minutes has passed.

Lean Arm Workout #2

This is a cycle workout, with a little change from those you have done before. You will be doing Arm Circles, as described below, to fill out the minutes of your workout, and you will march in place while you do.

Begin with 10 Plank Taps.

Do Arm Circles, while marching in place, to fill out minute 1. **Arm Circles** are done correctly this way:

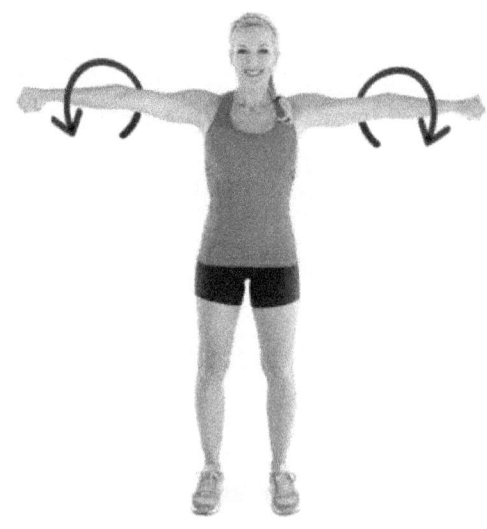

1. Stand up straight.

2. Keep your chest open, and your head up and forward.

3. Hold your arms out perpendicular to your body. Do not lock your elbows.

4. Move your arms in small circles, 3-5 inches, forward. You will reverse on the next cycle.

5. Remember to march in place at the same time.

When the timer reaches minute 1, do 10 Spider Lunges.
Finish minute 2 with Arm Circles, Reversed. Remember to march in place.

At minute 2, do 10 Pushups.

Complete minute 3 with Arm Circles, forward, marching in place.
When the timer reaches minute 3, do 10 Walkouts.
Fill out minute 4 with Arm Circles, Reversed, while marching in place.
Repeat these steps for the remainder of 15 minutes.

Lean Arm Workout #3

This workout is a cycle workout with Part A and Part B.

Part A

Begin with 10 of the Plank Arm Row and Rotate (Plank Arm R and R). The **Plank Arm Row and Rotate** exercise is safely and correctly accomplished this way:

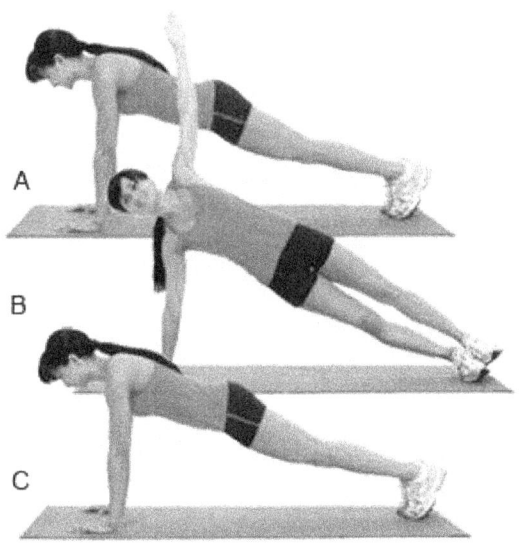

1. Begin in Plank Position.

2. Move your feet slightly wider than shoulder width apart.

3. Keeping your hips level and maintaining position, take your right hand off of the floor, and bend your elbow behind you to raise your hand up right next to your shoulder.

4. Return your hand to the floor.

5. Then, lift the same hand, with your arm bent, and rotate your torso so that your elbow is straight up in the air. Return your hand to the floor.

6. Repeat on your left side.

Rest 10 seconds.
Do 10 Pushups.
Rest 10 seconds.
Repeat Part A 8 times
Rest 1 minute

Part B

Do 10 Dip Kicks. **Dip Kicks** are performed this way:

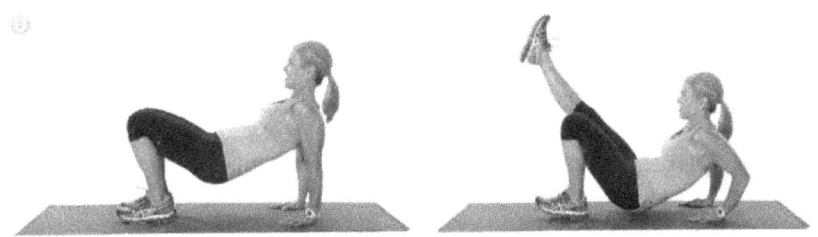

1. Sit on the floor with your knees bent, feet flat on the floor.

2. Lean your torso backwards about 45 degrees, while placing your palms on the floor, right under your shoulders with your fingers facing out.

3. Bring your left knee up towards your chest, and place your left foot on your right knee.

4. Bend arms directly behind you in a reverse pushup move, lifting your hips slightly.

5. Kick your left leg as you straighten your arms to come up.

6. Do all repetitions for this cycle on one leg. Remember to switch them on the next cycle.

Rest 10 Seconds.
Do 10 Walkouts.
Rest 10 Seconds.
Repeat Part B 8 times.
Rest 1 minute.

Cycle between Part A and Part B for the remainder of 15 minutes.

Lean Arm Workout #4

This is a circuit workout.

Start with 10 Pilates Presses. **Pilates Presses** can be done safely and correctly this way:

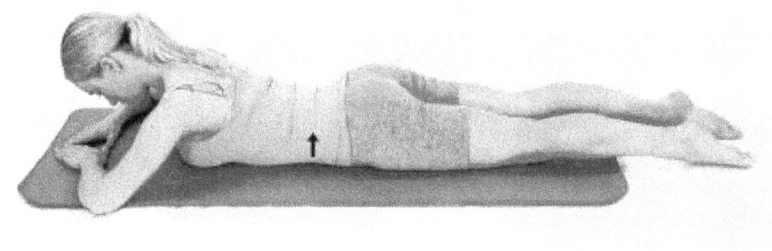

1. Begin in Plank Position. Remember to hold that position throughout the exercise.

2. Bend your right knee 90 degrees, pointing your toe towards the ceiling.

3. Bend your elbows directly behind you, keeping them close to your body, lowering yourself only a few inches. Do not try to go all the way to the floor.

4. Press back up.

5. Do all repetitions in this circuit on the same leg. Switch with the next circuit.

Rest 10 seconds.
Next, do 10 Dip Kicks.
Rest 10 seconds.
Do 10 Plank Taps.
Rest 1 minute.

Repeat circuit for the remainder of 15 minutes.

Lean Arm Workout #5

This is a cycle workout, with Part A and Part B.

Part A

Do 10 Full Circle Presses. Perform a **Full Circle Press** like this:

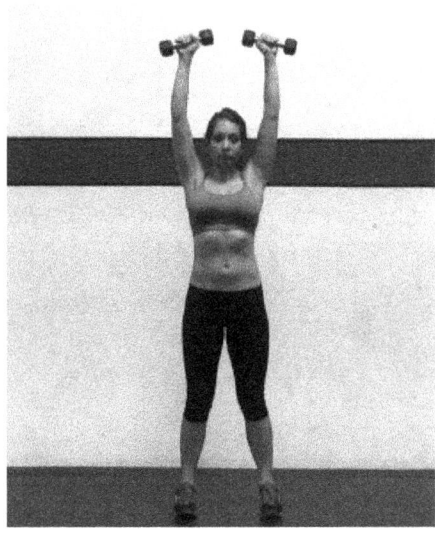

1. Begin in a Plank Position.

2. In one fluid, circular motion, shift your weight to your right arm, and begin lowering yourself towards the floor.

3. Lower yourself a few inches, then shift your weight across your body to your left arm.

4. Press back up.

5. Go in the same direction for one cycle, then switch the direction of your circle for the next cycle.

Rest 10 seconds.
Do 10 Walkouts.
Rest 10 seconds.
Repeat Part A 8 times.
Rest 1 minute

Part B

Start with 10 "X" Jumps. **"X" Jumps** are done correctly and safely in this fashion:

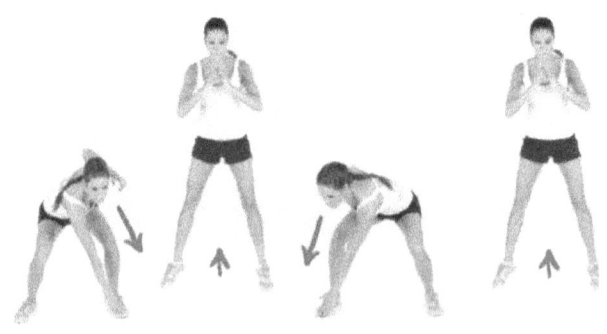

1. Begin in Plank Position, with arms directly below the shoulders, feet together.

2. Engage your core muscles and arms for stability.

3. Then, jump your legs out into a wide V.

4. Hop feet back together to complete the Jump.

Rest 10 seconds.
Repeat the cycle 8 times.
Rest 1 minute.

Continue alternating between Part A and Part B for the remainder of 15 minutes.

Others who are considering purchasing this book would love to know what you think. If you could spare a few seconds, they would greatly appreciate reading an honest review from you. Simply visit the page on Amazon..com.

Chapter 7

What You Should Eat

"Moderation in all things", an aphorism commonly ascribed to Aristotle, has been considered sage advice from Ancient Greece to modern times.

Nowhere is this more apparent than Western diet habits. Restraint, especially in the area of food intake, is difficult for all creatures, but none more so than human beings.

A Historical Perspective

Throughout our history, food was often scarce. People had to eat whatever was in front of them, right at that moment, or else it might be gone. This is a habit that has been passed on from parent to child for thousands of years.

More recently, The Great Depression caused food scarcity, and those who lived through that time taught their children to eat whatever was placed in front of them. Although that was many years ago, the repercussions of this practice are still being felt.

Why is this history important? Why should you care when you begin your own healthy eating plan? You should care because any adjustment of your habits begins in your mind, not your body. Recent diets play upon the human tendency to take everything to extremes. Combine this with the habit to consume vast amounts of food, and you have a recipe for disaster.

Everyone has heard stories of diets gone wrong, from removing too much fat and endangering the body's functioning, to restrictive types of vegan diets where proper nutrition is simply not possible.

The point here— "dieting" is difficult, and you are almost set up by history and biology to fail. While the 15 Minute Body Fix endorses a healthy eating plan, which you will learn about below, it is most important to keep it in perspective. Changing your life is not "all or nothing". A gradual process is best.

In other words, **do not** *beat yourself up if you are not instantly perfect at this!* Give yourself a chance to get the hang of it. After all, you are training your body to become stronger and more resilient. You have to fuel your body to accomplish this.

Low Carb vs. Low Fat

Food scientists debate which principle of dieting is best. Is lowering your fat intake the key to success, as you have been taught for years? Conversely, is the newer carbohydrate restriction method the most effective for weight loss and better health? The answer may surprise you.

Authority Nutrition recently compared a number of scientific studies on exactly this subject, and the results were clear. Not only did every group studied lose more weight on the low carbohydrate diet, but their bloodwork showed no ill effects from the inclusion of a moderate amount of healthy fats in the diet.

Low fat diets have a quicker effect on the blood markers for cardiovascular disease, but when compared again at a later time, the two diets were virtually equal. Healthier blood sugar readings, less hunger, and better cognitive functioning were all improved with the lower carbohydrate diet.

Each study had participants dropping out, because, as you have learned, "dieting" is hard! That is why you are going to focus on changing your habits. However, the lower carb, slightly higher fat diets seemed to retain subjects best. This is because fat helps keep you satisfied. You feel fuller and more nourished when you include some fat in your diet.

Fat Free for All?

So, you can really have all the fat you could possibly desire? Bring on the deep-fried cheese and keep it coming? Could that really be possible? Not exactly.

Remember the principle you learned at the beginning of this chapter. Moderation should be the basis of your eating plan. You will focus on carbohydrate reduction. However, trans fats and saturated fats have been proven to have some detrimental effects on the body, including the raising of so-called "bad" cholesterol which can lead to heart disease.

Still, monounsaturated and polyunsaturated fats actually raise the "good" cholesterol in your bloodstream and help you maintain cognition, and body function. As previously stated, they also help keep you satisfied.

Some Hints for Success

Some recipes are included later to give you some ideas of what to eat. You are also benefited by the current popularity of the lower carbohydrate diets.

However, you will benefit from a quick key to the foods you may want to avoid, and those you may want to include.

High Carbohydrate Foods to Limit

- Sugar, syrups, and sweeteners with calories
- Candies
- Dried fruits
- Boxed cereals
- Processed potato or grain-based snacks
- Cookies and cakes
- Jams, jellies, preserves and similar spreads
- Fruits in syrup
- Potatoes
- Bread
- Ice cream and frozen yogurt

"Bad" Fats to Limit

- Animal fats, including those in fatty meats and chicken skin
- Whole-fat dairy products
- Butter
- Stick margarine
- Packaged snack foods, like chips and crackers

- Deep-fried foods
- Most fast foods

As a guideline, total fat content in your diet should not exceed 20-35% of your total calorie intake. Limit saturated fats to less than 10%, and trans fats to less than 1% of your total daily calories

What *Can* You Eat?

At first glance, the list of things you should limit seems vast, but there are plenty of possibilities in the "plus" column. Generally, lean meats, vegetables, and fruits are on the menu. Fruits you will need to moderate to keep your carbs lower, but include them in moderation, because their health benefits are great. Low-fat versions of milk, cheese and other dairy products are acceptable, also in moderation. Nuts are excellent sources of protein, but are high in calories, which you must moderate if you want to lose weight.

Portion Control is the Absolutely Most Important Principle of Healthy Eating

Be aware of serving sizes. For example, the average small bag of nuts or trail mix that you might get at a convenience store will have 3-4 servings.

Organic foods have been proven to be higher in nutrition, due mostly to freshness. Speaking of freshness, look locally for the highest nutrition. Preparing food at home allows you to control your fats and portions easily.

Making the Best Choices

You will not always be able to eat at home. What do you do when you are out? How will you avoid sabotaging your entire plan? First of all, don't panic! Remember that you are not on a "diet", you are changing the way you eat. So, if your lunch isn't perfect, you haven't sabotaged anything! Wherever you are, make the best choice that is available. You know generally what to eat, and what to avoid. You can do this!

Many restaurants, even fast food places, now provide nutritional information for their food items to help you do this. If you don't see it, ask. Some people feel self-conscious when they do this, but your friends and family are going to see the healthier YOU being created. They will want to do what you are doing, so be proud to ask for what you need.

Again, **watch your portions,** especially if no nutritional information is listed. That is usually because you would not want to know! If you are confronted with a platter-sized plate, filled to overflowing with food, you know it is significantly more than you need. A common "dieter's" trick can come in handy with this. Ask for a box at the beginning of your meal, and place about half of what you see in front of you in it. Put it out of your eye line.

Getting Started

Often, when you first start a new eating plan, you need a little help! So, here are a few recipes that you may want to try for your low carb lifestyle.

Breakfast

Broccoli and Cheese Mini Egg Omelets

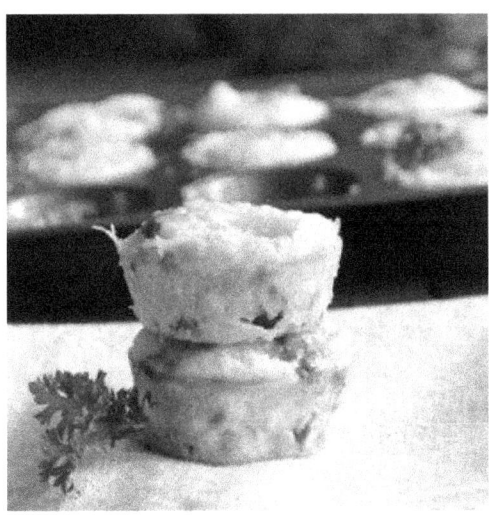

Ingredients

- 4 cups broccoli florets
- 4 whole large eggs
- 1 cup egg whites
- 1/4 cup reduced fat shredded cheddar
- 1/4 cup grated romano cheese
- 1 teaspoon olive oil
- Salt
- Pepper
- Cooking spray

Directions

1. Preheat your oven to 350 degrees. Steam the broccoli with a little water for 6-7 minutes.

2. When broccoli is well cooked, crumble it into smaller pieces, and add olive oil. Add salt and pepper to taste. Mix well.

3. Spray a standard sized muffin pan with nonstick cooking spray. Spoon broccoli mixture evenly into 9 tins.

4. In a medium bowl, mix egg whites, eggs, and cheese. Add salt and pepper to taste.

5. Pour the egg mixture into the muffin tins on top of the broccoli, until they are a little over ¾ full. You may add a bit more shredded cheese to the top once they are filled.

6. Bake in the oven until eggs appear solid, or cheese is crusty if cheese is added, around 20 minutes.

7. Serve immediately, two mini omelets per serving. These will also keep in the refrigerator for up to a week for quick breakfasts.

Savory Cheese and Chive Waffles

(For this recipe, you will need a waffle iron.)

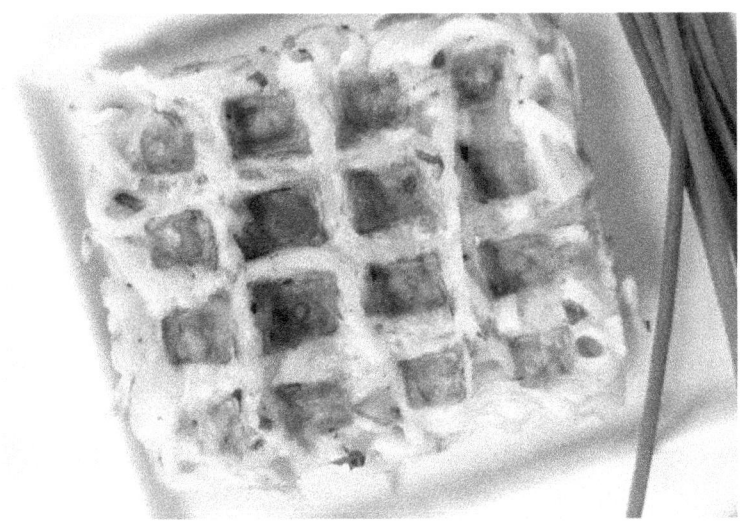

Ingredients

- 1 cup raw cauliflower chopped to the consistency of coarse crumbs
- 1/4 cup shredded mozzarella cheese
- 1/3 cup parmesan cheese
- 2 eggs
- 1 teaspoon garlic powder
- 1 teaspoon onion powder
- 1 tablespoon chives
- 1/2 cup sun-dried tomatoes (chopped to crumb consistency)

Directions

1. Mix well. Heat waffle iron. Fill iron with batter about ¼ full.

2. Cook 4-6 minutes. Iron will not stick when they are done. Serving size is one waffle.

Tex-Mex Scramble

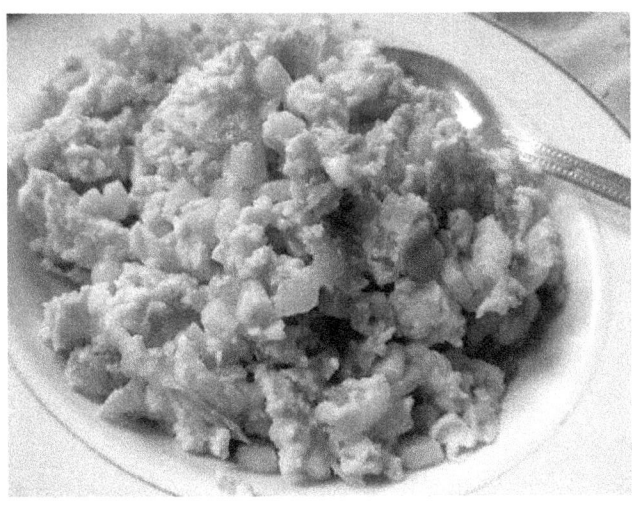

Ingredients

- 5 eggs
- 2 tablespoons water
- 1/8 cup chopped red onion
- 1/8 cup chopped green pepper
- 2 cherry tomatoes (diced)
- 1/2 cup frozen spinach (thawed and drained)
- 5 jalapeño pepper slices (chopped)
- 1 slice reduced fat pepper jack or cheddar cheese
- 2 tablespoons salsa

Directions

1. Preheat skillet over medium heat with canola oil (or healthy oil of your choice).

2. Mix eggs, water, onion, peppers, tomatoes, spinach and Jalapeños together.

3. Pour into oiled, heated skillet, and cook over medium heat until eggs are at your desired consistency.

4. Just before the eggs are ready to remove, add cheese to the top. Turn off the heat and cover eggs. Let stand 5 minutes. Add salsa to taste and serve.

Lunch

Bacon Wrapped Mini-Meatloaves

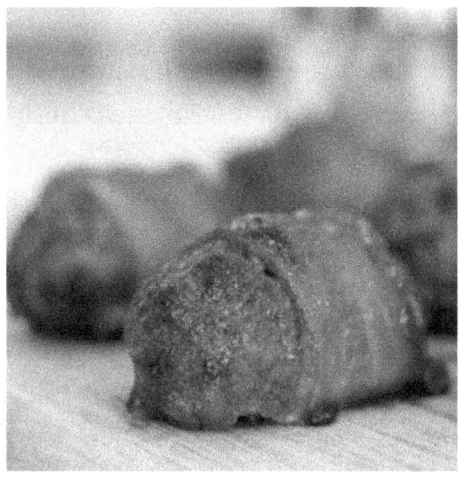

Ingredients

- 1 pound lean ground beef
- 1/2 pound bacon (cut into chunks)
- 8 additional strips of bacon
- 1/4 cup coconut milk
- 2 garlic cloves (minced)
- 1/3 cup fresh chives (minced)
- Fresh parsley (chopped)
- Freshly ground pepper to taste

Directions

1. Preheat your oven to 450 degrees.

2. In a big bowl, combine the ground beef, the bacon chunks, the coconut milk, the garlic, and the chives.

3. Mix well, until all ingredients hold together. You may use and electric mixer to save time.

4. Season the mixture with freshly ground pepper to taste. No need to salt, due to the saltiness of the bacon.

5. Take a medium sized muffin pan, and wrap a bacon slice around the inside of each tin.

6. Fill these holes with the beef mixture. Place in the oven and cook for 30 minutes.

7. Once cool enough to handle, remove and serve with fresh parsley on top. Serving size is one.

Bacon, Egg, Avocado, and Tomato Salad

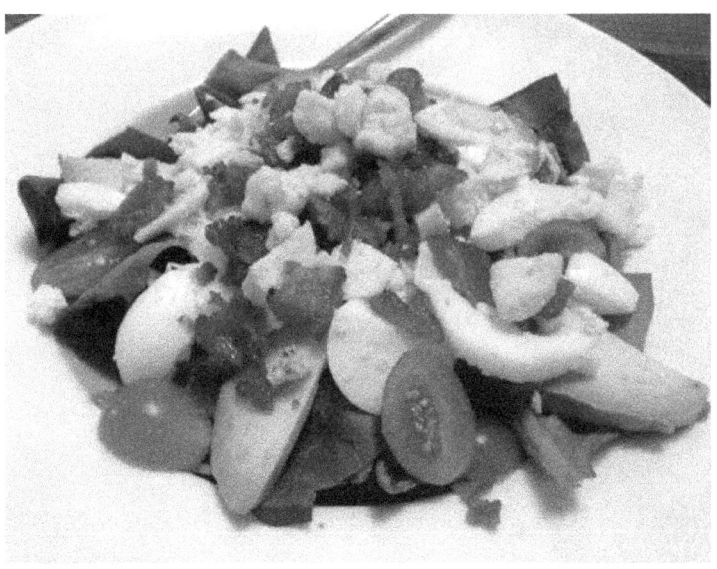

Ingredients

- 1 ripe avocado (cut into chunks)
- 2 boiled eggs (chopped into chunks)
- 1 medium-sized tomato (chunked)
- Juice from 1 lemon wedge
- 2-4 slices cooked bacon (crumbled)
- Salt and pepper to taste.

Directions

1. Mix all the ingredients together, not stirring too much, just until some of the eggs and avocado become mush.

Chef Salad Ham Cups

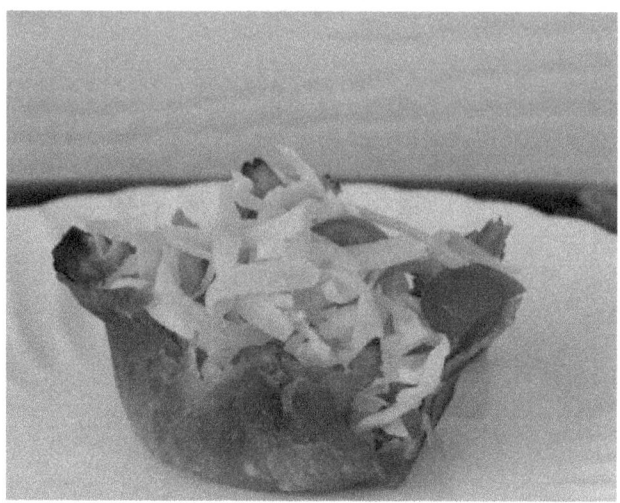

Ingredients

- 2 slices thinly-sliced ham
- Lettuce (chopped)
- Tomato (chopped)
- 1 hard-boiled egg (chopped)
- 1/4 cup cheddar cheese (shredded)

Directions

1. You will need 2 custard cups. Preheat oven to 350 degrees. Place 1 inverted custard cup on cookie sheet.

2. Place 2 slices of ham over the inverted cup, in an "X" formation for full coverage. Place 2nd custard cup over the ham to prevent shrinkage.

3. Cut excess ham from the bottom, leaving around 1.2 inches. Bake for 20 minutes. Place on cooling rack, and remove top cup to cool.

4. When cool, remove ham "bowl" from the bottom cup. Fill with lettuce, tomato, and egg. Top with cheese.

I hope you have learned something from this book so far and would greatly appreciate it if you could leave an honest review on Amazon.com.

Dinner

Crispy Carnitas

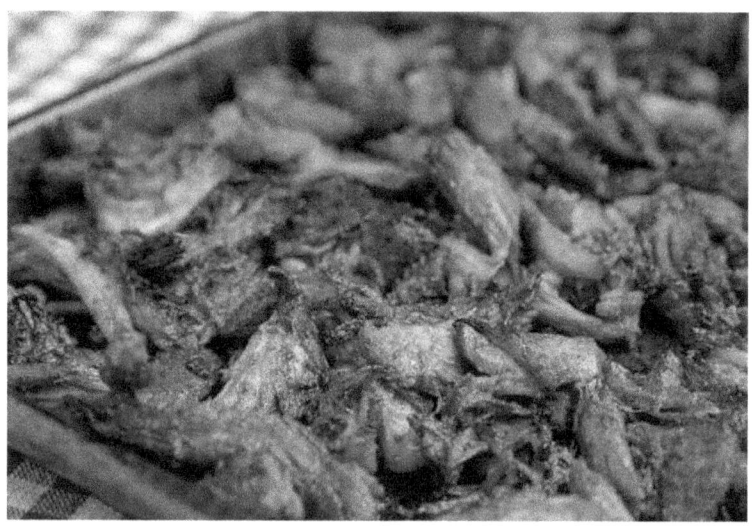

Ingredients

- 3-4 pounds of boneless pork shoulder (cut into 4-5 pieces)
- 1 1/2 teaspoons of salt
- 1 teaspoon cumin
- 1 teaspoon chili powder
- 1 cinnamon stick
- 1 bay leaf
- 4 garlic cloves (thinly sliced)
- 1 onion (chopped or thinly sliced)
- Water (for braising)

Directions

1. Preheat your oven to 350 degrees. Mix the salt, cumin, and chili powder together and rub all over the meat.

2. Place the meat in a single layer, in a large heavy pot, with the cinnamon stick, bay leaf, onion and garlic.

3. Add enough water to almost but not quite cover the meat. Put the pot in the oven and braise for 3-3½.

4. Stir the meat occasionally while it cooks. You will know the meat is done when it is tender and slightly browned. Most of the water will be gone.

5. Remove the pork from the oven, and then from the pot. Place it on your cutting board and shred it.

6. Remove the cinnamon stick and bay leaf from the pot. Return the shredded meat to the pot. Roast the meat until it is crispy. 1 cup is a serving.

7. Serve with green beans, snap peas, or asparagus.

Yellow Squash Casserole

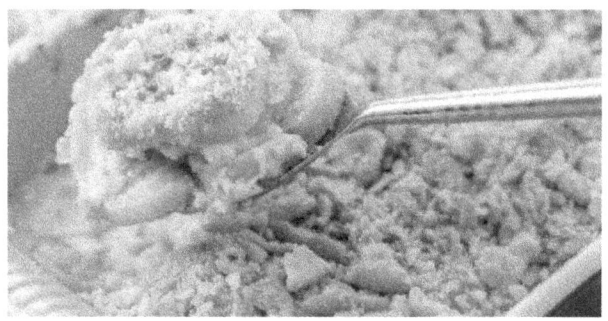

Ingredients

- 1 tablespoon olive oil
- 1 onion (chopped)
- 1 teaspoon butter
- 2 cloves garlic (minced)
- 1 teaspoon kosher salt
- 1/2 teaspoon of freshly ground peppers
- 4 cups yellow squash (cubed and peeled)
- 1/3 cup of raw almonds (chopped finely)
- 1/3 roasted (salted almonds, chopped coarsely)
- 1 cup colby-monterey jack cheese (shredded and divided in half)
- 1/2 cup heavy whipping cream
- 2 Eggs

Directions

1. Preheat your oven to 400 degrees. Heat olive oil and butter in a skillet over medium high heat.

2. Add garlic and onion, stir, and cook until soft, around 3 minutes. Add squash, salt, and pepper, stir to combine. Transfer squash mixture to a large bowl.

3. Mix raw almonds and a 1/2 cup of cheese into the squash mixture. Whisk cream and eggs together in a small bowl and add to the squash mixture.

4. Pour the squash mixture into a 9x13 inch casserole dish. Top with remaining cheese and roasted almonds.

5. Bake in oven until the casserole is golden brown and bubbling, approximately 25-30 minutes. 1/8 of the dish is a serving.

Pizza Frittata

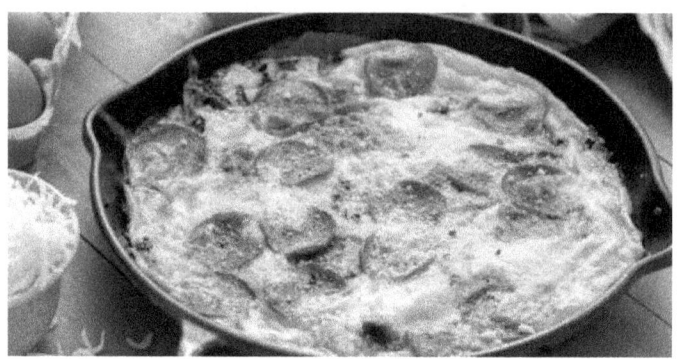

Ingredients

- 12 eggs
- 1 cup whole milk
- 1/2 cup grated parmigiano-reggiano cheese
- 1 teaspoon hot sauce
- salt
- pepper
- 1/4 cup of extra-virgin olive oil
- 1/4 cup pepperoni (finely chopped)
- 2 cloves garlic (chopped)
- 3 tablespoons grated onion
- 1 sprig of oregano (finely chopped)
- 1/4 dry red wine
- 1 cup crushed tomatoes
- 6 ounces of fresh mozzarella (grated largely, or sliced thinly)
- 1 small handful of flat-leafed parsley (chopped)
- A few fresh basil leaves (torn)

Directions

1. Preheat your oven to 400 degrees. In a large bowl, beat the eggs, milk, cheese, hot sauce, and salt and pepper to taste, until well mixed.

2. In a large, oven-proof skillet, heat 2 tablespoons of the extra virgin olive oil over medium to medium-high heat. Add the eggs, and keep moving and settling them as they cook.

3. When the eggs begin to firm up, transfer the skillet to the oven. Bake until golden and puffed, but not cooked through, approximately 10 minutes.

4. Meanwhile, in another, in another skillet, heat the remaining extra-virgin olive oil on medium to medium high heat. Add the pepperoni, garlic, onion, and oregano, and cook, stirring, for 2-3 minutes.

5. Add the wine; cook to reduce slightly, 1 minute. Then, add the tomatoes and simmer to thicken, around 10 minutes.

6. Remove the frittata from the oven, and top with the tomato sauce and mozzarella.

7. Bake to melt the cheese, another 8-10 minutes. Top with parsley and basil.

1/6 is a serving. Those are some ideas to get you started on your new healthy eating plan. Do remember, low carbohydrate eating is extremely popular- and you have learned why-so you will have many other options to try. Experiment and make eating fun!

Chapter 8

Top Tips for Success

Here are some tips to encourage you as you change your lifestyle with the help of the 15-Minute Body Fix.

Start Slowly

Remember that the workouts are meant to grow with you. Be realistic. If your fitness level is not what it should be when you start, modify them as suggested.

"No pain, no gain" is a misleading slogan. Your muscles will be sore after your workout, and you may have to concentrate on your breathing while engaged in it. However, if you experience severe pain while working out, or become extremely out of breath, you need to slow it down. You are meant to work up to this gradually.

Remember Your Rest Days

With the intense workouts you are doing, you need to let your body rest in between them.

As you start, you may only be able to work out 2 times a week. As you begin to feel confident, and are able to do the exercises correctly, add a day. 5 days a week is sufficient, according to experts. With routines like these, you need at least one rest day a week.

Additionally, do not concentrate on one area of the body for two days in a row. You could injure your muscles and set yourself back if you do.

Fuel Your Body

This may seem counterintuitive. However, your body is just like a machine, in that it needs fuel to run properly. Yes, your workouts will burn fat for fuel as they are intended to do, but you must also eat for proper nutrition.

Don't add to the meals you are already going to be eating. Instead, add a morning and/or afternoon heathy snack, such as celery with a serving of peanut butter or tuna, hard-boiled eggs, and single servings of nuts.

Watch your portion sizes, but include some protein. Protein knocks out that dizzy feeling better than anything else.

You will probably feel hungry until your body adjusts, which is perfectly normal. However, if you get dizzy between meals, that is like your car's gas light coming on. It indicates that it is time for a snack.

Do You Need Supplements?

If you are eating healthy foods, do you really need supplements? The answer is a resounding yes! There are essential vitamins and minerals that you will almost certainly be missing.

Be careful not to waste your money on supplements that do not give you the proper nutrition. Make sure your multivitamin gets its nutrition from food.

Chemically created vitamins do not work with your body correctly, and you will often flush most of them back out. Supplements derived from food are the only way to go. Check out your local health food store for options.

A good multivitamin should give you most of what you need, but including an extra Omega-3 supplement is a good idea. Also, if you are feeling low on energy, the B vitamins should be supplemented.

The Bs support your metabolism, and help you speed it up. Some people have a deficiency in this area and don't even know it, so if you are not feeling properly energized for your workouts, add some B-Complex to your life!

Do Not Forget to Hydrate

Water is essential to your body's functioning. The average person is made up of approximately 65% water. You will be sweating during your workouts. You need to replace that water!

8 cups of water a day in addition to anything else you drink is recommended. Other drinks do assist in hydration, but water does the job most efficiently.

Watch out for sneaky drink calories and sugars. Non-diet soda and sweet tea will not assist you in your goals. Soda in general is not as hydrating as other drinks because your body uses up some water trying to process the carbonation.

"Fitness" drinks generally have more calories than the average person needs to add to their diet. So, go with water instead!

Mix It Up

Fitness experts recommend switching out your workouts to avoid boredom and to keep you focused. This is why the 15-minute body fix gives you so many workouts to choose between.

Workout in the Evening

Many people like to get their workouts out of the way early in the day, but physical trainers suggest that you work out in the evening. Your body temperature is higher, which makes your workouts more effective.

Watch Your Neck

A mistake beginners often make is forgetting the correct head and neck positioning to avoid strain.

If you lift your chin too high, or tuck your head, you could hurt yourself. You should be able to fit a baseball between your neck and chin at all times during a workout. Imagine one there, and do not drop the ball.

Avoid Mirrors

Working out near a mirror is supposed to help your form. However, studies show that people who work out in front of mirrors feel more stressed and fatigued than those who don't.

Find Your Focus

It may sound funny, but experts say, think of someone who irritates you, then use that aggression in your workout. You can actually imagine your worries and cares being knocked out by your intense workout!

Listen to Music

Once you have learned your routines, some upbeat music will help you keep moving. Create special workout playlists of songs that make you want to move.

Don't forget to share your thoughts on this book by leaving a review on Amazon.com. It takes just a few seconds.

Discover Scientifically-Proven "Shortcuts" & "Hacks" to Lose Weight FASTER (With Very Little Effort)

For this month only, you can get Linda's best-selling & most popular book absolutely free – *Weight Loss Secrets You NEED to Know*.

Get Your FREE Copy Here:
TopFitnessAdvice.com/Bonus

Discover scientifically-proven tips to help you lose weight faster and easier than ever before. With this book, readers were able to improve their weight loss results and fitness levels. So, it's highly recommended that you get this book, especially while it's free!

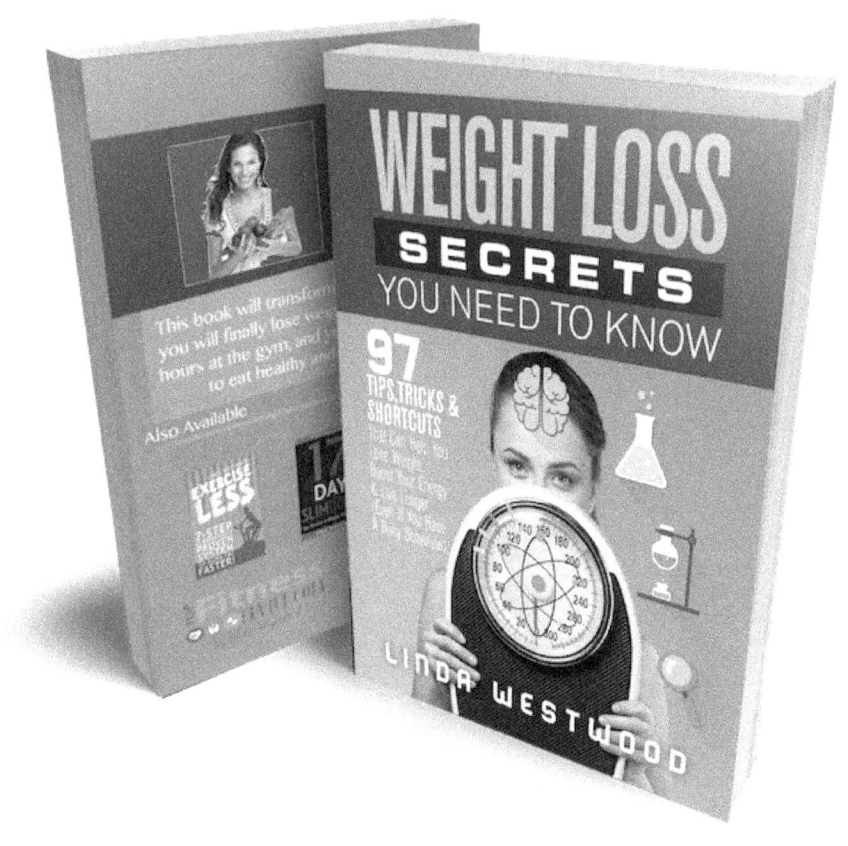

Get Your FREE Copy Here:
TopFitnessAdvice.com/Bonus

Conclusion

You have learned how important exercise is to your body. Physical fitness leads to health, improved cognition and a more cheerful state of mind.

You have also learned that exercise does not have to take half of your day. The 15-Minute Body Fix has shown you that you can tone up and lose weight in just 15 minutes a day.

You have the tools to accomplish this: amazing intense workouts that require nothing but you!

You know that healthy eating will help your workout's effectiveness, and you have a plan to help you learn to do just that.

You are ready to change your life with the 15-Minute body fix!

Final Words

I would like to thank you for purchasing my book and I hope I have been able to help you and educate you on something new.

If you have enjoyed this book and would like to share your positive thoughts, could you please take 30 seconds of your time to go back and give me a review on my Amazon book page.

I greatly appreciate seeing these reviews because it helps me share my hard work.

You can leave me a review on Amazon.com.

Again, thank you and I wish you all the best!

Enjoying this book?

Check out my other best sellers!

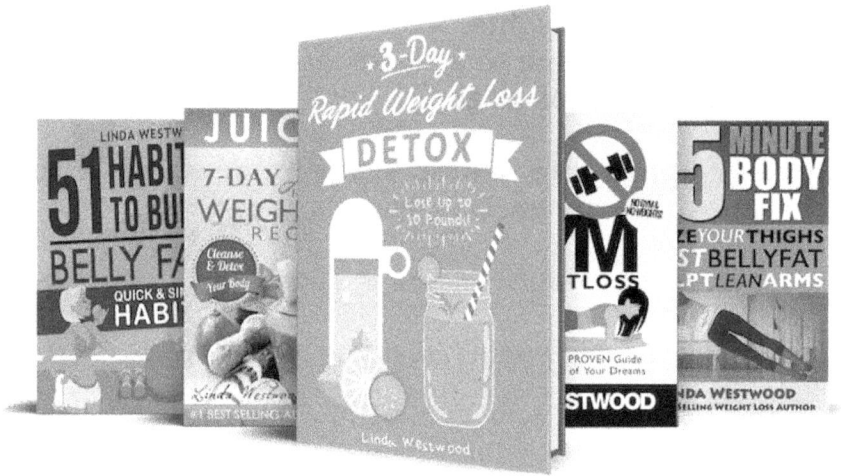

Get your next book on sale here:

TopFitnessAdvice.com/go/books

www.ingramcontent.com/pod-product-compliance
Lightning Source LLC
Chambersburg PA
CBHW031200020426
42333CB00013B/763